I Am Losing Weight

And Feeling Great

"Believe You Can And You Will"

A.J. Buonpastore

I Am Losing Weight

And Feeling Great

"Believe You Can And You Will"

I Am Losing Weight And Feeling Great

"Believe You Can And You Will"

Copyright © 2013 A.J. Buonpastore

"Believe You Can and You Will"

Dedicated To

Eleanor N Venturella Buonpastore

Contents

Introduction

What is it about human nature? We humans wrongly tend to believe certain things cannot be true for us simply because they are thought to be too easy to achieve. Believing that scenario to be valid is most unfortunate. I would like you to pause, stop reading and think for just a moment of what you just read. Think of why I have started this book with an introduction that implies that if you think, believe and desire certain things are too easy to achieve it just isn't going to be achieved, that it is impossible to be true because it is just too easy. My dear friend I am happy to say that you will find in reading this book that the complete opposite is true. Keep the idea above in mind as you continue to read through this book. The method that I suggest you use further on in this book is by far the easiest weight loss method known. Why isn't it advertised? Why haven't you heard of the easy method before? Why? Because no one makes any money, that's why.

"No other method on Earth is as easy and as powerful."

It's simple, believe that you can and you will. And guess what my friend; you can use my method for anything else that you would like to achieve. That's an extra bonus you get for buying my book.

You purchased this book because you want to lose weight, right? That is exactly what you will accomplish simply following my easy instructions further on in the book. Human nature is funny isn't it? We are so quick to believe that there are no easy solutions to some of our problems; it's got to be difficult or it won't work, duh, wrong! Maybe it's a stretch for me to make the statement above where I say; you can use my method for anything else you would want to achieve.

Allow me to clarify it so you understand what I really mean. Of course there are things nothing I say or that you can do will help. So let me add this little caveat to my statement; you can achieve most anything you want if you believe you can but it must be reasonable. That's the little kicker, it must be within reason, it must be reasonable. That's not so bad is it? You want to lose some weight; that's reasonable isn't it; you want to stop smoking; well that's reasonable, you want to grow to be 20 feet tall; nah, that's not reasonable and it's not going to happen. It's a silly example perhaps but I think you get the point.

Please don't get mad at me, I am not trying to be rude or a wisenheimer or a wise guy. You bought the book to help you lose weight and that's what you will accomplish. Let's face it you are overweight. How did you get there? I'll answer that for you; you ate too much and did too little. That is the simple truth.

But don't worry about it because you can change that if you really want to. Of course the best solution would be to stop eating as much and start exercising a lot; but that's not fun, is it?

Wouldn't it be fantastic if all you had to do to easily make important changes in your life was to follow a few simple instructions? Instructions that anyone can follow even a child. Just imagine what your new life would be like if you were able to make those changes anytime you wanted to make them.

You purchased this book expecting that it will do for you what it's advertised to do. Put your doubts away and let me assure you that you have purchased the easiest (a child can do it) the least expensive (there is nothing more to buy) and the most effective method ever created that anyone can use to lose weight.

Unlike most common weight loss books, systems, methods and programs that require special expensive diets, diaries, charts, carb watching, counting of calories etc. to work; you will be happy to find that the only requirement needed for my method to work for you is simply using the power of your subconscious mind; nothing more, nothing less.

I have wonderful news for you my friend; you can make any change in your life that you want just as long as the change you want to make is within reason. I will show you how to do it. You will lose the weight and you will feel great; that's a promise.

Yes you already possess everything you need to make changes in your life possible. You have within yourself an extraordinary power to make any change in your life you so desire. However (there is always a however isn't there) before you discover how to use this great extraordinary power you must make one very important commitment and that is simply to be honest with yourself; you must believe that you can. That's it in a nut shell. If you are honest with yourself and believe that you can, any change in your life that you really wanted to make simply becomes a matter of following a few simple rules and instructions that are clearly laid out for you in the following pages of this book.

I emphasize that you must be honest with yourself and believe that you can, because if you are not really being honest with yourself there is nothing in this world that can ever help you make any permanent changes to your life.

Okay, here is my promise to you; follow my simple rules and directions that I have provided for you in this book you will permanently make any and all the changes to your life that you really want to make, providing of course the things you want to change are within reason.

I could give you my methods and simple rules and instructions to follow here and now, but if I did, there wouldn't be much left for you to read. And you would probably put the book down and go away questioning if what I was writing about had any validity at all. So in the following pages I will do my very best to convince you to believe that making changes in your life isn't difficult at all. I will continue to write and fill as many pages as I can, not with boring fluff and fancy advertising claims and hype but with real facts.

We have all seen at least some form of advertising on TV, magazines, etc., each ad promising fantastic results. The product companies pay large sums of money to well known famous people to have them endorse and make questionable claims about their product. And of course they pass the cost they pay for their endorsements down to you added in the price of their products. We have seen the new TV Idol, or the movie star, or beautiful models wearing bikinis, or the world famous athlete etc., endorsing their products. We believe they are telling us the truth about the products they endorse. And so we buy the products that they recommend thinking the product will do whatever it is advertised to do.

We are constantly being bombarded in our daily lives with advertising, advertisers making extraordinary claims for their product to do one thing or another. In some ads of weight loss products the claims they make may be achievable providing of course you strictly follow their recommended agenda; which more often than not (especially of the weight loss programs) is eating healthy and exercising regularly. If you are a fast reader with super human eyesight you may be able to read the small printed text flashing across the bottom of your TV screen of most weight loss programs, stating that the examples shown are not typical, "oh really".

To take the weight loss ads discussion above a wee bit further let me add one other simple thought; "if we all ate healthy and exercised regularly as they recommend would we have a need for their products?" I doubt it. I am sure many of us would not have a need to use their weight loss program to begin with. That makes sense doesn't it?

Anyway, I will prove to you without any doubt the method provided for you within the pages of this book does indeed work. And can be used with great success by anyone who is serious and sincerely desires to make changes in their life.

The greatest thing about my method is you won't have to shell out a lot of money or follow any weird diet or eat foods that should only be eaten by grazing animals, count calories, or get your next meal delivered to you in a box, none of that nonsense.

And glory be, the changes you desire to make are not going to be limited to just weight loss; the changes you desire can be almost anything you want to change. The only prerequisite is that any change you want to make must be within reason.

"Believe You Can And You Will"

Chapter 1: The Magic of His Words

Before you begin to learn how to make the changes in your life that you desire I believe it is only proper for me to tell you with my deepest respect and admiration for the man that the method you are about to learn in part was first originated by Émile Coué 1857–1926; a French Chemist, Psychologist and Pharmacist who introduced a popular method of psychotherapy and self-improvement based on optimistic autosuggestion.

He was world renowned in his time for curing thousands of patients suffering from a myriad of illnesses using his self improvement method. He is also noted for having the distinction of coining the popular phrase; "Every day, in every respect, I am getting better and better".

He was not only famous for curing his own individual patients, but also taught others in various facets of the medical profession how to use his method for curing their patients as well.

Working as a Pharmacist, he quickly discovered what is known as the placebo effect. What is the placebo effect?

A definition of placebo effect: A written prescription for a patient that contains no real medicine, it is given for the positive psychological effect it may have simply because the patient believes that he or she is receiving treatment.

Another definition of placebo effect: Something of no inherent benefit that is done or said simply to placate or reassure somebody.

He became known for reassuring his clients by praising each of his prescribed remedy's efficiency and leaving a small positive notice with each given medication.

He noticed that in certain cases he could improve the efficacy of almost any given medicine by praising its effectiveness to the patient. He realized that those patients to whom he praised the medicine had a noticeable improvement when compared to patients to whom he said nothing. Thus, these observations were to become the beginning of his exploration in the use of the power of autosuggestion.

A definition of autosuggestion: The process by which somebody's perceptions, behavior, or physical condition may be altered by means of his or her power of suggestion.

At first, his method for treating patients relied on hypnosis. He then discovered that subjects could not be hypnotized against their

14

will and that the effects of hypnosis waned quickly after the patient regained consciousness. He then turned to the power of autosuggestion, which he described as; an incalculable mind force that all humans possess at birth.

He believed in the effects of medication. But he also believed that our mental state is able to affect and even amplify the action of these medications. By consciously using autosuggestion, he observed that his patients could cure themselves more efficiently by replacing their "thought of illness" with a new "thought of cure".

According to his method, repeating words or seeing images enough times causes the subconscious mind to absorb them. The cures of his patients and subjects then were the result of their subconscious minds accepting and using imagination or "positive autosuggestion".

He thus developed a method which suggests the principle that an idea that occupies the mind exclusively turns into reality. Of course the idea must be practicable and within reason.

An example would be if a person suffered from headaches such as migraines, firmly believes that his or her migraine is disappearing, then this may actually happen. However, if a person was born without a leg at birth, it would be unreasonable to expect a leg to grow.

It is reasonable to expect that our subconscious mind has the power regardless of the illness in our body to physically overcome or control the illness. Furthermore, thinking negatively about the illness; "I am not feeling well" will only serve to encourage both mind and body to accept this thought.

In 1913, Émile Coué and his wife founded The Lorraine Society of Applied Psychology. His book Self-Mastery Through Conscious Autosuggestion was published in England (1920) and in the United States (1922). Although Coue's teachings were, during his lifetime, more popular in Europe than in the United States, many Americans who adopted his ideas and methods, such as Norman Vincent Peale, Robert H. Schuler, and W. Clement Stone, became famous in their own right by spreading his words. The list of names above is but a small sampling of believers. I too have adopted his belief.

However, his method of autosuggestion takes a more general approach to healing the body. Therefore if there were more than one affliction it would require more time to heal because the subconscious mind is not concentrated on any particular one of them. Whereas in using my method the results are realized much, much faster because my method directs the subconscious mind to deal only and directly with one problem at a time.

"Believe You Can And You Will"

Chapter 2: The Power

Émile Coué was not alone in his thinking that a force of great power exists in every human being. Many scholars, mental and physical medical professionals, are also in agreement, that this extraordinary force most certainly exists, though some may have and do give alternative names and descriptions to it.

There are many simple experiments that you can do to prove the power does exist. We do these simple experiments on a daily basis without ever realizing we are doing them.

For example you are fast asleep but suddenly awakened because you feel a need to go to the bathroom or you might be warned of an odor of something burning or you may feel the presence of someone hovering over you, etc. If you are asleep how can this be? Who, why or what is warning you of the impending danger you may be about to discover? The above is merely a small fraction of functions that the subconscious mind has control over. Adding to that are all of your bodily functions including your digestive system, respiratory system, etc.

The power I am referring to cannot literally be seen in our brain. But that is where it resides. Our brain as it is called has many functions. Most importantly it has two very distinct minds. Let me repeat that again so you won't think I made a typo. Every human has one brain, every brain has two minds. The names given to the two minds are "Conscious Mind" and "Subconscious Mind" they reside in the brain.

To answer the question above as to Who, Why or What is warning you of impending danger; it is the subconscious mind; it stands guard and gives warning to the sleeping body while the conscious mind is at rest. While both minds are powerful it is the subconscious mind that controls every function in our bodies.

The subconscious mind is an extraordinary force with incalculable power. Convince the subconscious mind that you believe something to be certain then, whatever that something is, it becomes a reality. Thus the saying or quote: "You are what you think you are".

Within the pages of this book you will learn how to easily teach yourself a simple and powerful method when used properly convinces your subconscious mind to develop and bring about the reality of wants and desires you may have; even though you may now think they are impossible. Grasp the simple idea above and you will be well on your way to becoming the master of your body.

"Believe You Can (Lose Weight) And You Will".

Understanding the concept of Conscious and Subconscious Minds is of vital importance to your success in achieving your goals. I will continue to repeat myself at the risk of redundancy to the importance of your belief in the power of the subconscious mind. Please forgive me for being redundant but I am doing it because I want you to succeed and in order for you to succeed you must believe in the power of your subconscious mind.

It is also very important that you remember too, the subconscious mind without control is free and often does meander. If you were to continually feed it verbally and visually with negative thoughts, images and suggestions it responds in kind with negative results. So from here on in you must cease to think negative thoughts. From here on you will be the most positive person anyone and everyone loves and knows.

"Believe You Can And You Will"

Chapter 3: The Method...

Programming The Subconscious Mind:

In this chapter you will learn how to program your subconscious mind. By now I am sure you've got the idea. Convince (program) the subconscious mind to do what you want and it becomes a reality. The subconscious mind is always busy taking care of the body's natural functions and learning new ones as we age and progress in life. Some of the natural functions are programmed and preset at birth. Others are from learned experiences gained through the use of our five senses.

A good analogy would be a computer. When a computer is first purchased it usually comes with a hard drive and a few preset programs; then you continually add programs to it to make it function in the way you want it to. Such is the subconscious mind. Your subconscious mind needs to be programmed before it can bring about a wanted and desired action.

The subconscious mind is more powerful than any computer ever built; it is the most powerful entity in the universe. Programming your subconscious mind is by far much easier than trying to program a computer. Those of you with any experience would know that writing a computer program of any significant value is difficult.

Programming the subconscious mind is nothing new. The practice of doing so has been going on for quite a long time. Its use throughout medical history is well documented. Many well-known practitioners have written hundreds of books and thousands of pages about this very subject.

The practice and experiments continue to this day in secret military and clinical laboratories throughout the world in secluded unmarked or disguised clinics and institutions. The methods used and the names that are given to these experiments are kept secret.

The term brainwashing I am sure is familiar to many. The results of brainwashing are brought about by the use of repetition, deprivation, torture and reward. Remember the experiments of Pavlov and the dog?

The methods used in this book are simple to learn, they are completely safe and require nothing more than the repeated utterance of words and the optional use of a mechanical means (the counter string of knots) to bring about a desired benevolent result.

The net expected results are wholly dependent upon the total belief given to the method by the individual participants.

There are many ways to program the subconscious mind. We will discuss just two methods that anyone can use to program their subconscious mind. They are through verbalization (saying and hearing) and visualization (writing and seeing); that's it. You will learn how to easily do both.

Let's start with using verbalization. Returning for a moment to Émile Coué, whose famous mantra; "Every day in every way I am getting better" was the key to the great success he had in healing thousands of patients and clients. In his modesty he believed that he did not heal anyone, only taught them to heal themselves. How true that statement is, simply because it is your body and only you can control what you do with it.

The method is simple, easy to apply and very successful and has been ever since he created it.

The verbalization of a mantra; what then is a mantra? (A mantra is an expression or idea that is repeated, often without thinking about it, and closely associated with something). The association for you is losing weight.

I will suggest a simple mantra (an expression) that you can use. It is not by any means chiseled in stone; you can create your own if you wish. The idea of the mantra is to program the subconscious mind into producing the results you desire from the words you are saying. When the subconscious mind is filled with only your one thought (the idea of your mantra) the subconscious mind will transform your thought into reality.

A couple of points to remember is, (one) your mantra should only refer to one idea at a time; (two) repeat your mantra in a manner as though it has already been achieved, using a monotone voice.

For best results use the mantra at least three times a day, in the morning when first awakening, at noon in a comfortable chair and at bedtime repeating the chant at least twenty times during each session. Your eyes should be closed and without thinking about anything else; repeat the mantra as many times as possible but try for at least twenty.

Mantras are used by many cultures; they are often used with the use of a place holder made of a string of beads. It helps keeping the mind concentrated on the mantra and assists in the counting. I personally used a strand of leather with twenty knots tied onto it. It really did the job and faster than I thought it ever would.

The mantra I have created for you is simple and to the point. Use it if you like it, or create your own. Try to keep it as short as possible but by all means it must convey your true desire to the subconscious mind. Remember what I said about the manner to which you speak, make it sound as though what you expect to occur is already a reality.

Below is the mantra I have created for my readers that wish to lose weight...It is also the title of this book...

"I'm Losing Weight And Feeling Great".

I think my first example above is fantastic, it's short, it's positive, and it will certainly accomplish your goal of losing weight.

Example...

"I'm Losing Weight And Feeling Good"

Example...

"I'm Losing Weight And Getting Thin"

Example...

"I'm Getting Thinner And Looking Good"

Listed below to help you succeed and in no particular order are additional simple instructions and examples of mantras for you to use. Some of which may be repeated from above.

Instructions on how to communicate with the subconscious mind to achieve maximum results are very simple; some critics and non-believers will even think they are childish but I assure you they are not and the reality of your desired results will be proof enough.

It is extremely important that the mantra be repeated at least twenty times. Using the mantra counter assures mechanical recitation.

And now you will learn how to communicate with and consciously implant ideas through repetitious suggestions into the subconscious mind with the use of a simple mantra of words.

Every night before going to sleep and every morning before rising and anytime during the day or evening that is convenient while lying in bed or sitting comfortably on a chair, without noise or distraction from any source close your eyes, relax and in a low murmuring voice and tone as if you were reciting a prayer or a mantra, using a mantra counter repeat with confidence no less than twenty times consecutively the mantra below; repeat it over as often as you can.

The use of the mantra counter assures mechanical recitation, which is very important.

While articulating the mantras words don't think of your weight or any of your troubles. Be passive with the desire that all will be for the best. Be relaxed, have confidence in yourself. You will recite the mantra without effort. Feel as though your desires will be realized and they will be realized sooner or later. Have faith and firmly believe that all will be well.

I AM, are two very powerful words; there can be no doubt as to who they refer to. Using the words I AM (losing weight) repetitiously in the mantra will bring about positive results.

"I am Losing weight and it is easy"

"I am going to lose weight, I am going to lose weight, I am going to lose weight," (repeat 20 times).

For a powerful general statement that can be all inclusive and does not address any one specific need you may wish to use the following:

I AM getting better everyday in everyway!

It is very similar to the mantra that the famous chemist "Emile Coue" used to cure thousands of patients with varying afflictions, both physical and mental. His famous mantra is as follows:

"Everyday in every respect I am getting better and better"; repeated 20 times or as often as possible with the help of a knotted string to assure mechanical recitation.

Select the phrase you want as your desired result and repeat it as often as possible. Make use of the mantra counter whenever you can to assure a minimum repetition of at least twenty times.

What is most important is the recitation and repetition of simple words with the belief that the results are imminent and soon to be realized.

"Believe you can and you will"

"By believing oneself to be the master of one's thoughts one becomes what he thinks".

"Become the master of your SHIP, your bodily domain".

"Everyone of our thoughts, good or bad, materializes and becomes in short a reality".

Caution, do not use the word "Will", it invokes the idea of will power. Will power can be your enemy; let me explain. Have you ever tried to recall something you have forgotten, perhaps the name of an old friend that you haven't seen for quite a while; the more you try to recall the name the harder it gets to remember. It's because your subconscious mind isn't cooperating with you. However if you relax and say something like it's okay it's been awhile since I last saw this person, I'll recall his or her name in a moment or two; then sure enough the name pops into your head. The same often occurs with students taking a test; they have studied hard and know the answer but for the present moment it eludes them, the harder the student tries, the harder it becomes to remember. If the student lingers on at the question trying to will the answer to come to mind, it won't.

If the student goes on to the next question or two without trying to invoke his will power to remember, the answer to the question he or she could not remember comes to mind. What really is happening is that the use of will power is being applied to the subconscious mind; i.e.; I will remember the name or I will remember the answer. If the subconscious mind is not in agreement with whatever you are willing it to do, whatever it is, it's not going to happen. Quite possibly an opposite action most likely occurs.

By using the method I have described for you above you can easily make any changes to

29

your being you so desire as long as the changes you want to make are reasonable. You must be practical as well and not expect any change to happen overnight. Be patient, give it time and know that the change you seek is going to become a reality. Changes in some people occur more quickly than in others, but be assured the changes will happen. If you are on any prescribed medication continue to do so, do not make any changes without consulting with your physician. As the saying goes "Rome wasn't built in a day" and that also applies to your body. Take your time and know in your heart and mind you are going to make the change you desire. You are going to lose weight.

We have discussed in detail above one of the two methods that can be used to program your subconscious mind. The verbal method is easy, very powerful and convenient; all that one needs to do is continually repeat a set of words that form an idea, commonly called a mantra. Visualization is the other method I referred to earlier. Of the two methods "visualization" is the more powerful of the two; however, on the other hand, it is not as easy or convenient to practice.

Visualization of course requires images, producing an image that can represent your desire is awkward and impractical. When I refer to images, your first thought I am sure would be to think of producing photographs or pictures of some type, not necessarily so; it can be an image of some text written on paper and the method would be to repeat the written text hundreds of times.

Many years ago when I was in elementary school I remember the teacher telling me to write a sentence 100 times on the blackboard. I was told to do so as a punitive means to remember not to chew gum in class. Well needless to say, I never chewed gum in any classroom again.

Visualization is a very power method. Using this method would probably result in realizing your goals much quicker. I doubt however if many would have the time and patience to use this method. But by all means if time isn't a problem please use it. Just use the same mantras indicated above. Write it and repeat writing the line at least twenty times. Write it as often as you can; three, four, five times a day, more if you can. Do not let anyone discourage you. Don't pay attention to any ridicule from anyone; in fact use it to your benefit. As I indicated above don't expect overnight results, be patient. Seeing is believing; the more often you write and see your mantra the faster your subconscious mind will respond.

"Believe You Can And You Will"

Chapter 4: The Minds Of Believers

I thought it fitting to include in this book, interesting observations made over time by many different people who are in agreement that the subconscious mind is a powerful entity that can be used to bring action and reality to our thoughts.

Below are a few thoughts of my own:

Why not use the all-powerful forces of your mind as nature intended and gives to all human beings at birth! It's your life and you are the only one that can bring about a desired beneficial and permanent change.

Redirecting your mind is easy using a simple method of repeating a set of words; i.e., a mantra.

When you control your subconscious mind, you become the master of your ship.

So capable and all-powerful is the subconscious mind it can bring about realities to desires you presently may think are impossible, they become a reality if you believe they can and they are reasonable.

James Allen wrote a wonderful book titled:

"As a Man Thinketh". The title is influenced by a verse in the Bible from the Book of Proverbs chapter 23 verse 7, "As a man thinketh in his heart, so is he" in his body."

James Allen: From poverty to power:

The most powerful forces in the universe are the unseen forces—the silent forces; and in accordance with the intensity of its power does a force become beneficent when rightly directed, and destructive when wrongly employed.

This is common knowledge in regard to the mechanical forces, such as steam, electricity, and the like, but few have yet learned to apply this knowledge to the realm of mind, where the thought-forces, most powerful of all, are continually being generated and sent forth as currents for salvation or for destruction

When the thought-forces are directed in harmony with the over-ruling law, they are constructive, up-building and preservative, but when subverted they become disintegrating and self-destructive.

To adjust all your thoughts to a perfect and unswerving faith in the omnipotence and supremacy of good is to cooperate with that Good, and to realize within yourself the solution and the destruction of all-evil. Believe.

Show me a man under whose touch everything crumbles away, who cannot retain success even when placed in his hands, and I will show you a man who dwells continually in those conditions of mind, which are the very negation of power.

To be forever wallowing in the bogs of doubt, to be drawn continually into the quicksand's of fear, or blown ceaselessly about by the winds of anxiety, is to be a slave and to live the life of a slave, even though success and influence be forever knocking at your door seeking for admittance.

Such a man, being without faith and without self-government, is incapable of the right management of his affairs, and is a slave to circumstances, in reality a slave to himself. Such are to be taught by affliction, and ultimately to pass from weakness to strength by the stress of bitter experience.

Whatever your position in life may be, before you can hope to enter into any measure of success, usefulness, and power, you must learn how to focus your thought-forces by cultivating calmness and repose.

It may be that you are a businessman suddenly confronted with some overwhelming difficulty or probable disaster. You grow fearful and anxious, and are at your wit's end.

To remain in such a state of mind would be fatal, for when anxiety steps in, correct judgment passes out.

Now if you will take advantage of a quiet period in the early morning and at night, go to some solitary spot or to some room in your house absolutely free from intrusion, and, having seated yourself in an easy attitude, will forcibly direct your mind away from the object of anxiety by dwelling upon something in your life that is pleasing and bliss-giving, a calm, reposeful strength will gradually steal into your mind and your anxiety will pass away.

On the instant you find your mind reverting to the lower plane of worry bring it back again, and re-establish it on the plane of peace, poise and power. When this is fully accomplished, you may then concentrate your whole mind upon the solution of your difficulty, and what was intricate and insurmountable to you in your hour of anxiety will be made plain and easy, and you will see with that clear vision and perfect judgment belonging only to a calm and untroubled mind, the right course to pursue and the proper end to be brought about.

It may be that you will have to try day after day before you will be able to calm your mind perfectly, but if you persevere you will accomplish it.

And the course, which is presented to you in that hour of calmness, must be carried out.

Doubtless when you are again involved in the business of the day and worries again creep in and begin to dominate you, you will begin to think that the course is a wrong or foolish one; but do not heed such promptings.

As you succeed in gaining mastery over your impulses and thoughts you will begin to feel growing up within you, a new and silent power, and a settled feeling of composure and strength will remain with you.

Your latent powers will begin to unfold themselves, and whereas formerly your efforts were weak and ineffectual, you will now be able to work with the calm confidence that commands success.

Along with this new power and strength will be awakened within you that interior illumination known as "intuition," and you will walk no longer in darkness and speculation, but in light and certainty.

With the development of this inner vision, judgment and mental penetration will be incalculably increased, and there will evolve within you that prophetic vision by the aid of which you shall be able to sense coming events, and to forecast, with remarkable accuracy, the result of your efforts. In just the measure that you alter from within will your outlook upon life alter; and as you alter your mental attitude towards others they will alter in their attitude and conduct toward you.

As you rise above the lower, debilitating, and destructive thought-forces, you will come in contact with the positive, strengthening, and up-building currents generated by strong, pure, and noble minds, whereby your happiness will be immeasurably intensified, and you will begin to realize the joy, strength, and power that are born of self-mastery alone.

"A man's foes are they of his own household," and he who would be useful, strong, and happy, must cease to be a passive receptacle for the negative, beggarly, and impure streams of thought; and as a wise householder commands his servants and invites his guests, so must he learn to command his desires, and to say, with authority, what thoughts he shall admit into the mansion of his soul.

You have the power of choice; so, turn on the light and develop the positives, and the negatives or darkness shall disappear. Even a very partial success in self-mastery adds greatly to one's power, and he who succeeds in perfecting this divine accomplishment, enters into possession of undreamed of wisdom and inward strength and peace, and realizes that all the forces of the universe aid and protect his footsteps who is master of his soul.

If you are given to fear, anger, worry, jealousy, greed, or any other inharmonious state of mind, and expect perfect physical health, you are expecting the impossible, because you are continually sowing the seeds of disease in your mind. Such conditions of mind are carefully shunned by the wise man, for he knows them to be far more dangerous than a bad drain or an infected house.

If you would be free from all physical aches and pains, and would enjoy perfect physical harmony, then put your mind in order, and harmonize your thoughts.

Think joyful thoughts, think loving thoughts, let the elixir of good will course through your veins; you will need no other medicine. Put away your jealousies, your suspicions, your worries, your hatreds, your selfish indulgences, and you will put away your dyspepsia, your biliousness, your nervousness and aching joints.

If you will persist in clinging to these debilitating and demoralizing habits of mind, then do not complain when your body is laid low with sickness.

Christian Daa Larson: Thinking for results:

Man is as he thinks and his thoughts are invariably created in the likeness of his mental conceptions of those things of which he thinks about habitually.

Therefore as man improves his mental conceptions of all things he will improve himself in the same measure.

To improve these mental conceptions attention should always be concentrated upon the ideal of everything of which we think. That is, all thinking should move toward the greater, the larger and the superior.

Whatever we think about we should always think about its ideal side, its larger side and its superior side.

Everything has two sides, the limited or objective side and the unlimited or subjective side. When we consider only the limited objective side of those things we think about our mental conceptions will be small, superficial and materialistic.

When we think about ourselves we should always think about the unlimited possibilities of the within. Attention should be directed upon the larger self, and every thought should be formed in the likeness of the highest mental conceptions that we can form of the superior.

We may, however, recognize the existence of flaws in our nature; in fact, it is necessary to know where the weak places are in order to remove them; but the mind should never hold its attention upon those weak places. The mental eye should never look upon the imperfect, but should look through it and direct its vision towards the ideal.

And here we find the reason why the average person does not improve as he should. The fact is he thinks of himself as he appears to be in the limited personal self. He patterns his thought after the small life that he can see in the outer self.

And as man is as he thinks he will therefore not rise above the quality or the nature of his own thought. No one can rise any higher than his thoughts. Therefore, so long as your thoughts are like your present limited personal life you will never become any more than you are now.

The mind, however, that transcends its present states, talents and qualities and tries to gain mental conceptions of the larger and the superior will steadily rise and become as large as those new conceptions that have been formed, and may later rise still higher thus

40

reaching greater heights of consciousness, ability, and power than was dreamed of before.

In the world of feeling the thorough application of the law of scientific thought is extremely important, the reason being that we generally live upon those planes where our feelings are the strongest.

All our feelings therefore should be transformed to the highest planes of thought and living that we can possibly think of. But since feelings deal principally with forces, whether in mind or personality, it is in the world of force that we shall have to direct our attention if a change of feeling is to be made.

And very simply training the mind to always try to feel the finer and the more powerful forces that are back of every state, condition or action does this.

Whenever anything takes place in your system try to feel the finer forces in that part of the system where the action is taking place. This experience may not give you any new sensation at first, but you will gradually become conscious of a whole universe of finer life and action within yourself. Then your mind will be living in a much larger world and in a much richer world.

These finer life forces that you feel within yourself are the powerful creative energies of the subconscious, and it is these energies that are so valuable in the development of the mind and the reconstruction of the body. Therefore, whenever you exercise the sense of feeling try to feel the higher and the finer that is in you.

You will soon succeed and the results will not only add enjoyments, both to mind and personality, but will also give you the mastery of new and powerful forces.

An expanding and ascending desire should be back of every action of the mind, and all efforts to gain the conscious realization of the new should aim at the very largest mental scope and realization possible.

Every desire should desire the largest, the purest, the most refined and the most perfect expression that present mental capacity can be conscious of. This will add remarkably to the joy of living and will have a refining effect upon the entire system.

The most refined expressions of desire give the greatest pleasure, whether the channel of expression is physical, mental or spiritual. But no desire should be destroyed. The proper course is to refine it and turn it into, channels through which the forces back of that desire can be wisely employed now.

When we refine our desires those desires will never lead us into wrongs or temptations because the fact is that a refined desire never desires to do wrong. On the contrary, every desire that desires higher and higher expressions will, through such a desire, tend to enter into the right, the more perfect and the superior.

In this connection, we should remember that all ascending actions are right actions, that all descending actions are wrong actions, and that this is the only difference between right and wrong.

Every mental aim should have the greater in view, and every plan that is formed should embody the largest possibilities conceivable. Too many minds fail because their plans are so small and their aims too low; but the larger and the higher is invariably the purpose of scientific thought-thought that thinks for results.

Every mental force, therefore, should be an aspiring force and should have the power to spur us on to greater efforts and higher goals. This is extremely important; as we shall know when we learn that all forces are creative.

When all the forces of your system are trained to aspire, everything that is being created in your system will be created more perfectly and you will steadily advance.

Christian Daa Larson: How the mind works:

The principal reason why the average person remains weak and incompetent is found in the fact that he makes no effort to fathom and understand the depths of his real being. He tries to use what is in action on the surface, but is unconscious of the fact that enormous powers are in existence in the greater depth of his life.

These powers are dormant simply because they have not been called into action, and they will continue to lie dormant until man develops his greatest power; that is, the power to discern what really exists within him.

The average person lives on the surface. He thinks that the surface is all there is of him, and therefore does not place himself in touch with the live wire of his great and inexhaustible nature within. He does not exercise his greatest power the power to discern what his whole nature may contain, and therefore does not unlock the door to any of his other powers.

This being true, we can readily understand why mortals are weak. They are weak simply because they have chosen weakness. But when they choose power and greatness they shall positively become what they have chosen to become. And we all can choose power and greatness, because it is in us.

44

William Walker Atkinson:" Thought-force in business and everyday life:

We are all influenced much more than we are aware by the thoughts of others. I do not mean by their opinions, but by their thoughts. A great writer on the subject very truly says: "Thoughts are Things." They are things, and most powerful things at that.

Unless we understand this fact, we are at the mercy of a mighty force, of whose nature we know nothing, and whose very existence many of us denies. On the other hand, if we understand the nature amid laws governing this wonderful force, we can master it and render it our instrument and assistant.

Every thought created by us, weak or strong, good or bad, healthy or unhealthy, sends out its vibratory waves, which affect, to a greater or lesser extent, all with whom we come in contact, or who may come within the radius of our thought vibrations.

The casting in of a pebble like the ripples on a pond causes thought waves; they move in constantly widening circles, radiating from a central point. Of course, if an impulse projects the thought waves forcibly toward a certain object, its force will be felt more strongly at that point.

Besides affecting others, our thoughts affect us, not only temporarily, but also permanently. We are what we think ourselves as being. The Biblical statement that "as a man thinketh in his heart, so is he," is literally correct.

We are all creatures of our own mental creating. You know how easy it is to think yourself into a "blue" state of mind, or the reverse, but you do not realize that repeated thought upon a certain line will manifest itself not only in character (which it certainly does), but also in the physical appearance of the thinker.

This is a demonstrable fact, and you have but to look around you to realize it. You have noticed-how a man's occupation shows itself in his appearance and general character. What do you suppose occasions this phenomenon? Nothing more or less than that thought.

Action follows as the natural result of vigorous thinking. You think in earnest, and action does the rest. Thought is the greatest thing in the world.

Now, I am going to change that "I Can't" into a big "I Can".

Good thought attracts other good thoughts; the bad thoughts, the bad; thoughts of strength, likewise; thoughts of discouragement and doubt follow the rule, and so on through the entire gamut of thoughts.

Your thought attracts to it the corresponding thoughts of others and increases your stock of that particular kind of thought. Do you see the point? Think fear thoughts, and you draw to yourself all the Fear thought in that neighborhood. The harder you think it, the greater supply of undesirable thought flocks to you.

Think "I am Fearless," and all the courageous thought force within your radius will move towards you, and will aid you. Try it.

Don't think Fear thoughts. Do you know that Fear and its oldest child, Worry, are at the bottom of more misery, more unhappiness, and more failures, than anything else in the world? Fear and Hate are the parents of all the vile thoughts.

Tear them out by the roots. They spoil the whole garden and breed hosts of other weeds, such as Worry, Doubt, Timidity, Lack of Self Respect, Jealousy, Spite, Malice, Envy, Slander and Morbid Ideas.

If you were my dearest friend, and I knew that this message would be my last on earth, I would shout to you, as loud as my vocal organs would permit: "Let Go of Fear and Hate Thoughts!"

Fenwicke Lindsay Holmes: "The law of mind in action"

The subjective or subconscious mind, therefore, is found to control the involuntary functions of the body such as the beating of the heart, the contraction and expansion of the lungs, and the digestion of food; we do not have to think consciously about these things; they are done unconsciously.

The important fact about the subconscious mind is this: it is the builder of the body, or the creative mind. Under its direction new life cells are constantly being born to take the place of those, which have finished their work and are passing away.

New heart cells are born each minute, new lung cells, new nerve tissues. As every action consumes energy and thus produces waste in the system, the subconscious mind must busy itself with carrying away the waste through the blood, pores, kidneys, lungs, and waste system, and at the same time go about to build new life cells to take the place of the old.

Thus a marvelous activity is constantly going on within us, asleep or awake, of which we are entirely unconscious; and a million servants of

48

the system are each scurrying to his appointed place to do his workman-like task.

So it is literally true that "every day is a fresh beginning, every morn is the world made new," for we rise with a renewed body which is so frequently reconstructed that every organ and tissue is doubtless born anew in the course of one year or less.

All these procreative agents are very susceptible to mental attitudes and reflect our thought either for health or disease. For example, the blood is known to contain certain agents for the destruction of dangerous germs (a germ being an objectified disease thought).

These agents customarily approach the foreigner, encircle him, literally cover him with sauce to make him palatable and proceed to eat him. But if the individual is mentally depressed and negative, the little guardian of the body reflects his attitude, does not cover the germ with sauce and refuses to eat him. Then trouble ensues. This scientific fact shows the Bible to be correct when it says, "As a man thinketh in his heart, so is he" in his body.

Prentice Mulford: Your forces:

There are two kinds of age, the age of your body, and the age of your mind.

Your body in a sense is but a growth, a construction of today and for the use of today.

Your mind is another growth or construction millions of years old. It has used many bodies in its growth. It has grown from very small beginnings to its present condition, power, and capacity in the use of these many bodies. You have, in using these bodies, been far ruder and coarser than you are now.

You have lived as now you could not live at all, and in forms of life or expression very different from the form you are now using; and each new body or young body you have worn has been a new suit of clothes for your mind; and what you call "death" has been and is but the wearing out of this suit through ignorance of the means, not so much of keeping it in repair, as of building it continually into a newer and newer freshness and vitality.

That power is your thought. Every thought of yours is a thing as real, though you cannot see it with the physical or outer eye, as a tree, a flower a fruit.

Your thoughts are continually molding your muscles into shapes and manner of movement in accordance with their character.

If your thought is always determined and decided, your step in walking will be decided.

If your thought is permanently decided, your whole carriage, bearing, and address will show that if you say a thing you mean it.

If your thoughts are permanently undecided, you will have a permanently undecided gesture, address, carriage, or manner of using your body; and this, when long continued, will make the body grow decidedly misshapen in some way, exactly as when you are writing in a mood of hurry, your hurried thought makes miss-happen letters, and sometimes miss-happen ideas; while your reposeful mood or thought makes well-formed letters and graceful curves as well as well-formed and graceful ideas.

You are every day thinking yourself into some phase of character and facial expression, good or bad. If your thoughts are permanently cheerful, your face will look cheerful.

If most of the time you are in a complaining, peevish, quarrelsome mood, this kind of thought will put ugly lines on your face; they will poison your blood, make you dyspeptic, and ruin your complexion; because then you are in your own unseen laboratory of mind, generating an unseen and poisonous element, your thought; and as you put it out or think it, by the inevitable law of nature, it attracts to it the same kind of thought-element from others.

You think or open your mind to the mood of despondency or irritability, and you draw more or less of the same thought-element from every despondent or irritable man or woman in your town or city.

You are then charging your magnet, your mind, with its electric thought-current of destructive tendency, and the law and property of thought connects all the other thought-currents of despondency or irritability with your mental battery, your mind.

If we think murder or theft, we bring ourselves by this law into spiritual relationship and rapport with every thief or murderer in the world.

Your mind can make your body sick or well, strong or weak, according to the thought it puts out, and the action upon it of the thought of others. Cry "fire" in a crowded theatre, and scores of persons are made tremulous, weak, paralyzed by fear. Perhaps it was a false alarm. It was only the thought of fire, horror acting on your body that took away its strength.

The thought or mood of fear has in cases so acted on the body as to turn the hair white in a few hours. Angered, peevish, worried, or irritable thought affects injuriously the digestion.

A sudden mental shock may lose one's whole appetite for a meal, or cause the stomach to reject such meal when eaten. The injury so done the body suddenly, in a relatively few cases, by fear or other evil state of mind, works injury more gradually on millions of bodies all over the planet.

If you expect to grow old, and keep ever in your mind an image or construction of yourself as old and decrepit, you will assuredly be so. You are then making yourself so.

If you make a plan in thought, in unseen element, for yourself, as helpless, and decrepit, such plan will draw to you of unseen thought-element that which will make you weak, helpless, and decrepit. If, on the contrary, you make for yourself a plan for being always healthy, active, and vigorous, and stick to that plan, and refuse to grow decrepit, and refuse to believe the legions of people who will tell you that you must grow old, you will not grow old. It is because you think it must be so, as people tell you that make it so.

If you in your mind are ever building an ideal of yourself as strong, healthy, and vigorous, you are building to yourself of invisible element that which is ever drawing to you more of health, strength, and vigor.

You can make of your mind a magnet to attract health or weakness. If you love to think of the strong things in Nature, of granite-mountains and heaving billows and resistless tempests, you attract to you their elements of strength.

If you build yourself in health and strength today, and despond and give up such thinking or building tomorrow, you do not destroy what in spirit and of spirit you have built up.

That amount of element so added to your spirit can never be lost; but you do, for the time, in so desponding, that is, thinking weakness, stop the building of your health-structure; and although your spirit is so much the stronger for that addition of element, it may not be strong enough to give quickly to the body what you may have taken from it through such despondent thought.

Persistency in thinking health, in imagining or idealizing yourself as healthy, vigorous, and symmetrical is the cornerstone of health and beauty. Of that which you think most, that you will be, and that you will have most of.

You say, "No." But your bed-ridden patient is not thinking, "I am strong;" he or she is thinking," I am so weak." Your dyspeptic man or woman is not thinking, "I will have a strong

54

stomach." They are ever saying, "I can't digest anything;" and they can't, for that very reason.

The mood of mind you are in on first arising is the mood most likely to last during the day. You may not feel the growth of more courage, decision, or even temper from this simple practice, at first.

You will in time; and you will wonder at the change in yourself, and where your greater force, courage, decision, or other good healthful thought came from. If you call this trivial, ask yourself if you know anything at all of the nature or cause or composition of a single one of your own thoughts.

You are very apt to carry the hurried mood of mind in which you tie your shoestrings into the writing of a letter which may involve to you the gain' or loss of thousands of dollars. The hurried, impatient mood runs its wire of disorderly thought and slovenly act straight through from one act to another, and leaves its traces and its damage on all.

And so when you have dressed in a hurry, eaten in a hurry, and rushed to the street car in a hurry, if you do not carry hurry and neglect and forgetfulness into your business, you may still have the harder task to throw off this mood of mind, and get "into the more reposeful and deliberate one in which you pursue your business or occupation; and in trying to get down to your work, or, in other words, get up that interest and enthusiasm or enjoyment in your work, which you crave, and without which you cannot do it, you use up a great deal of force which might have been put directly in your work, and which you might the sooner have had, had you laid for it the cornerstone by tying your shoestrings with a religious and devout carefulness in the morning, and in so doing have connected a religious, careful, orderly, and therefore pleasant and profitable mood of mind to every act done throughout the day.

It pays in dollars and in health and in happiness to make well-formed letters in writing, for the mood, which makes the well-formed letter, begets the mood, which makes the well-formed plan.

And, although you may see men apparently successful who are always in a hurry, you will find on closer examination theirs is not a whole success; for, though they may gain in wealth of dollars, they are surely losing in the wealth of health, without which nothing that dollars bring can be enjoyed.

That is not a healthy mind or body, either, which can enjoy nothing but the heaping up of money, the article which represents food, clothes, shelter, and all necessary and enjoyable things.

The slower movement of body which characterizes the religious form, rite, and ceremonial of all faiths, and in all ages, had for its object, and was intended by a greater Wisdom as a first lesson, to teach man the use and profit and pleasure which comes of putting our thought, or as much thought or force as may be necessary, on the act we are doing now.

It is law of our beings, that, when the painter can put his whole thought in the handling of his brush; when the orator or actor puts his whole force on his method of expression, and allows none of that force to stray off in the self-conscious channel of thinking how A, B, or C may judge or criticize that method; when, as Shakespeare says, you give to each proportioned thought its act (that is, carry out the act as your thought has first shaped or planned such act), as when the athlete or gymnast or graceful dancer put their whole thought or force in the muscle needed for use, and expression at the instant, there comes of this the careful religious concentrative mood or use of our force, always bringing pleasure to ourselves and pleasure to others; and the giving first of happiness to ourselves, and next happiness to others, through the proper use and expenditure of the forces belonging to us, is the great aim and use of the sentiment or quality we term religion.

Every impatient act, no matter how trivial, costs an unprofitable outlay of force or thought. Every impatient act is an act without a plan. You do plan a blow with a hammer before you make it: if you did not, the hammer would strike wide of its mark. You plan the proper intonation or accent of a word before you speak it. You plan the graceful movement before you make it.

These things may be planned with the quickness of lightning or thought, but planned they are; and those acts bring pleasure to you and others from being well done. That is the reward of mental temperance, and there are much greater rewards, also; for the habit of so doing all acts brings you more and more power and health and strength.

When you tug impatiently at the knob of the door that won't open easily, or pull impatiently at the knot that won't untie, you are sending force or thought into that knob or knot with little or no plan as to its use or direction. You are sending, also, a great deal more force or thought into that knob or knot than is needed to open or untie.

This is an intemperate use of force. This is the wildest extravagance, because it is expending force you cannot recall, in effecting nothing. It is expending far more power than if it had been deliberately planned, not only uselessly so far as this effort is concerned, but

58

you are strengthening the habit of so uselessly expending or wasting force in the doing of all things.

You are training your mind to this habit of extravagance, and this habit will bring you weakness and loss in every direction.

When you send your thought or force ahead of your body, and in the store toward which you are hurrying (as you actually do while hurrying to that store), the most of your real and invisible self goes to that store, and is in that store, uselessly expending itself, because it has not the body, its instrument, to work with.

It has not the body's senses to touch with, the body's physical eye to see with, and the body's material tongue to talk with. You are really in that store, having only your finer or interior senses, and these cannot act on material things.

You are then as a carpenter would be who came to his work without his saw or hammer or other tools. Your thought, your invisible self, or most of it, in the store represents the carpenter. The saw or hammer represents your body, which you are dragging wearily on, with the little spirit or force left in it, five or six blocks away; and the force you expend uselessly, In dragging it, could have been better used in selecting the proper quality of cloth, or matching colors, or in seeing that you did not have some article forced upon you by the salesman, who knows just what you want, because you haven't mind enough left in you, when you've got your body at last in that store, to know what you want yourself.

Force means judgment and tact and discretion and taste; you know your part, temporarily, with most of these qualities when you are hurried and flurried and flustered and excited. It is when in this condition, that the salesman, who is cool and collected, and has all his wits, his force, his thought, about him, can throw his mind or thought into yours, and make you see with his eyes, and judge with his judgment; and as a result you may buy what you find, on getting home and pulling yourself (your mind) together, that you don't want it at all.

It is this habit of mind, which causes what is called "nervous diseases." When you send your thought, or force, away from your body to some place you are hurrying the body to, be it store, railway station, ferryboat, or the top of the stairs, you are sending away from you that unseen element of strength for which the nerves are the conductors through your body, as the telegraph-wire conducts from town to town a cruder form of the same force.

When you fall into the habit of sending it away, you are tremulous, or, as we say, the nerves are shaken, for lack of this unseen vital power. Sudden fright may send instantly a great volume of this element from you.

Hence the body has no strength left in it. In other words, your real self, your spirit, your force, has mostly gone from the body; and, when fright kills, it is because an actual end or link of unseen element, which bound spirit and body together, has snapped. Your invisible self is really an organized body of this force.

The more nerve or force you call to the body, or any part of the body, you would use, the more nerve you will have. The more nerve you get, the more you will attract to you. There is no limit to its increase. Your thought or force so by habit set massed in a bunch, as it were is a magnet, ever growing in power to attract more force.

Orison Swett Marden: How to get what you want:

Faith moves mountains.

"To him that believeth, all things are possible." The man who does not believe in something and believe in it with all his soul is a pretty poor stick. (old English for unfortunate)

61

Let nothing undermine your faith in your ultimate triumph. Hold this tenaciously, vigorously, intensely, and after awhile you will see things coming your way.

Don't be afraid to think too highly of yourself. If the Creator made you and is not ashamed of the job, certainly you should not be. He pronounced His work good, and you should respect it.

Faith increases confidence, carries conviction, and multiplies ability. Faith doesn't think or guess. It sees the way out. It is not discouraged or blinded by mountains of difficulties, because it sees through them—sees the goal beyond.

There are marvelous utilities, infinite good and unspeakable beauties in the great cosmic intelligence, the unseen world, ready for our use and enjoyment. If we only had sufficient faith to believe they were there we could draw them to ourselves.

Writing of heroes discovered by the world war, Edmund Kemper Broadus says: There is no philosophy, no power in the universe that can help me to do a thing when I think I can't do it.

More people make wrecks of their lives from lack of faith in themselves than from any other cause. There is only now and then a man who really believes in his own bigness, who has sufficient faith to back up his ability.

And ability must be backed up by a superb self-confidence before it can accomplish anything. The ability of a Napoleon or a Webster would be absolutely powerless without self-confidence.

Before we can win out in life we must believe in our power to win. We must be confident in our expectations of success, vigorous in our self-faith. We must believe in ourselves and the things we are doing, without reserve and with all our hearts.

Ralph Waldo Trine: The higher powers of mind and spirit:

We are all dwellers in two kingdoms, the inner kingdom, the kingdom of the mind and spirit, and the outer kingdom, that of the body and the physical universe about us. In the former, the kingdom of the unseen, lie the silent, subtle forces that are continually determining, and with exact precision, the conditions of the latter.

To strike the right balance in life is one of the supreme essentials of all successful living. We must work, for we must have bread. We require other things than bread. They are valuable, comfortable, but necessary.

63

It is a dumb, stolid being; however, who does not realize that life consists of more than these. They spell mere existence, not abundance, fullness of life.

"Believe You Can And You Will"

Chapter 5: Food For The Mind

Thoughts ~ Belief ~ Desire

Thoughts:

What is a thought? The dictionary defines "thought" as the activity or the process of thinking. I think it should also mean to thinking in the past tense; or referring to an idea that occupied your mind at one time.

It's important to know that thoughts or what you think is one of the key elements that communicate to the subconscious mind what you want it to do for you; because if you don't think about it, it can't happen. In fact nothing happens unless you think about it, elementary, rudimentary yes simple but very true. Nothing ever happens to you in your life unless you think about it. As long as you and I are alive we will always be thinking of something.

To communicate with the subconscious mind you must constantly think of what it is you want it to do. Thinking however is just one of three elements needed to impress upon the subconscious mind an idea. Unfortunately just thinking of an idea you want to impress upon the subconscious mind is great but isn't quite enough to have it materialize. You need to really desire it with all your being to make it

65

happen. You are getting close to seeing your desire become a reality but before you can you need one more very important element and that is belief. It is a combination of these three very important elements when used together forms the key that unlocks the powerful forces of the most extraordinary entity in the world, you subconscious mind. The elements are your Thoughts, your Belief and your Desire.

The following are some of my thoughts about, well, about thoughts. Thoughts have wings and fly, not real wings of course, they are invisible and travel very fast perhaps at the speed of light or faster if that were possible. If it were possible to see thoughts traveling they would resemble the ripples of water in a lake or pond after a stone or some object was dropped into it, the ripples or waves emanating out in every direction from the point the object was dropped into the water. Another example would be like a radio or a television signal being transmitted out from a transmitter tower.

Since thoughts have no mass they can easily pass through solids made of almost anything. They pass through your brain and the walls of your skull; they pass through the walls of your building and into space. They travel continuously without ever stopping traveling round and round, new thoughts as well as old thoughts mixing together. There are three parts to our thought making system all of which are controlled by the mind.

A thought receptor, allows us to receive thoughts. A thought generator allows us to create and send our thoughts. A thought filter allows us to separate thoughts.

Fortunately for us nature has provided human beings with thought receptors. The thought receptors are somewhat mysterious and unknown to many in the modern medical and scientific community. The thought receptor quickly examines thoughts as they pass through our minds, then hands off thoughts to the thought filter for further examination. The thought filter decides whether or not a thought would be of interest to the force.

If I were asked where and in what part of the human anatomy are these thought receptors, generators and filters I would say they are of course in your mind and are a part of our brain. Where else could they be?

Although there are times when I have listened to the thoughts of others and seriously wondered what part of their anatomy their thoughts were really coming from.

Thinking or having one thought at a time becomes a challenge to most of us and is sometimes difficult to do because we are constantly bombarded with thousands of thoughts passing through our mind at any given moment sent out into the atmosphere continuously by humans the world over.

We separate the jumble of unclear and clouded thoughts from the continuous bombardment of other thoughts by the use of a thought filter. When we choose to further zero in on one particular thought we make use of a filter and then focus in on that particular thought. Thus, when we focus on one thought at any one time it becomes clearer and more meaningful.

Try this experiment; try to think of one thing, anything at all for a few moments. Your mind is immediately filled with extraneous thoughts unrelated to the subject you wish to think about. However if you concentrate on the subject you have chosen and stay focused by eliminating all extraneous interference you will then have a clear thought of the subject you have chosen. Try it.

Another example of what I call the reverberation of thoughts is; this has happened to me on more than one occasion; many years ago long before the idea was invented or ever used I thought about placing video cameras on the dashboards of police vehicles. Seriously, I knew the technology existed and it wouldn't be at all difficult to put together a proto type and then convince police and public safety departments to buy into my idea.

Well needless to say I did nothing except tell my wife and family about my idea who agreed it was a good idea. But unfortunately like so many other ideas that often come and go I did nothing.

Shortly afterward the police vehicle dashboard camera was born and it now is a tremendous tool for police departments all over the world. Was it really my idea or did I get the idea from someone else's thoughts? I don't know for sure and it's for sure I will never know.

Where did I get the idea? I never had any associations with electronics firms or police departments. Where did the idea come from in the first place?

I believe it came from the minds of many people that were thinking about and probably working on that idea. But the credit and rewards will go the person or people who stayed focus on the idea and brought it to the market place.

How many times has that experience happened to you? At least a few times I bet. How many times have you encountered something new and said to yourself I thought about that? Or how many times have you said I wish I had thought about that? How many times have you said I have a great idea and did nothing more about it? If you were to ask me that question my answer would certainly be many, many times. Perhaps next time a good idea comes along we will act upon it.

If it were possible for you to see the invisible atmosphere that surrounds all of us (known sometimes in parapsychology as ether) you would see billions and billions of waves of ideas and informational thoughts, emanating from the minds of billions of humans; thoughts about everything possible and thoughts going in every possible direction.

I did say earlier thoughts have no boundaries. Thoughts form in everyone's mind then travel outward in every direction at the speed of light without control or guidance without ever stopping, nothing stops a thought, and it can penetrate almost anything never bending or curving and travel into outer space; eventually becoming universal thoughts.

Billions of thoughts are generated twenty four hours of every day by billions of human beings. They pass through our minds at the speed of light.

Fortunately for us our thought receptors have a built in mechanism, they are called filters, the entire thought processing system is controlled by the subconscious mind and as part of the thought receptors process we are able to filter through the bombardment and conglomeration of thoughts that pass through our minds and hold onto a particular thought if the subconscious mind feels that a certain thought may be of interest to us. I am sure you have heard the phrase, "hold that thought".

Thought receptors and thought filters are controlled by our subconscious mind and knows from experience what is and what is not of interest to us as individuals.

In this chapter we have discussed and learned a little something about thoughts. We learned thoughts emanate from the minds of every human being on earth. We also learned that thoughts travel outward in concentric circles like ripples in a pond having no boundaries and that they can penetrate solid objects with impunity.

We also know that thoughts are the product of thinking. We determined that you cannot think without creating a thought. They are synonymous. They are the same. When you are asked what are your thoughts on a particular subject you are really being asked what are you thinking.

Thinking is the first rule and one of the three elements everyone must have and use if a positive outcome is to be expected from the subconscious mind. You must think clearly of the action you want before your demands given to the subconscious are to be expected as a positive result.

To be successful in anything you must continuously "THINK" about it, and want it with all your heart and soul and believe that you will and can achieve it. There is so much to say and discuss about the subject of thoughts. I will leave most of the discussion for another time.

Belief:

What is belief? Webster's dictionary says; Assent of the mind. I wasn't sure I liked that definition so I decided to look up believe and it said "to expect with confidence" ah hah! That's much better I thought.

And so this is as good an explanation of belief as I could conjure up without going to extremes. Belief is the act of believing in something without having doubt.

If you believe in anything at all you must first believe in yourself. Please remember this statement, it is very important.

Without belief how could you reach your goals, how would you succeed in anything, well, you wouldn't and you couldn't. Believing is the belief you put into your thoughts to make them become a reality. But first believe in yourself.

Don't worry or stress yourself out about failing if you wanted to try to do something. If you have ever failed trying to do something, or if things didn't turn out the way you expected, it's no big thing, everyone fails at one time or another; just pick yourself up, dust yourself off and start all over again, (that line also comes from a song).

Failure is not the end of the road; it is merely a temporary roadblock. Correct your errors and start over again. Seldom do we reach our desired goals on the first try.

Isn't it reasonable to say if you didn't believe in what you were doing whatever you were doing would not be worth while? If you didn't believe in whatever you were doing you would just be going haphazardly through the motions to get it done and it would not be your best work or accomplishment and perhaps even turn out to be a failure.

On the other hand if you did believe in what you were doing no matter what the undertaking, you would do your very best work and accomplish the feat with amazing results. And so it is with most things in life. We do great things in life when we believe that we can.

Belief is a fundamental, necessary element that you must inject into the subconscious mind. It is necessary that you believe in order for the subconscious mind to bring about your expected results.

When we believe in something it is without doubt and without question. The feeling it mentally gives to us is strong and unshaken and nothing can change our feeling.

Don't be dismayed or distracted by others who may say it won't work or your wasting your time, they say it out of ignorance, they say it because they know it is much easier to quit without reaching your goal than to start over and try again.

Stay firm and focused on your goals. Success may be just one more try away. Believe you can succeed and you will.

The world is full of pessimistic and doubtful people. I call them the non-achievers. They go through life like so many sheep in the meadow. Never wanting more than what the sheep rancher has provided for them, water and a handful of grass; satisfied with the status-quo not knowing or wanting anything more.

I wonder though if the sheep would act the same if they knew what the future held for them. Well, the sheep don't have any choice nor do they possess intelligence so maybe that's not a fair comparison to make. Most of us humans do have a choice and hopefully some intelligence, we are not sheep. We make our own decisions in life. We decide what we are going to do with our lives.

And unlike sheep and the non-achievers some of us want more from life than the status-quo, water and grass, because we are the achievers.

To reach beyond the status-quo we set goals for ourselves reaching higher and higher, never satisfied always attempting to do better. This is the idea that makes life so wonderful, always trying to set higher standards, always trying to accomplish the impossible, always inventing new ways and different things and always doing what others say can't be done and accepting the challenges.

This is the life I want to live and I know this is the life you want to live as well, or you would not be reading this book, we do not want to live the mundane life of a sheep. My friends it can be yours, you can live your life to the fullest, it is here for you to take don't be discouraged by the negative chants of those who live the status-quo. Set your goals, believe in yourself, believe you will achieve your goals and I promise, you will.

75

Desire:

What is desire? We know from the dictionary that it means the eagerness to obtain or enjoy. And it can also mean to wish for the possession or enjoyment of. There are a couple of other meanings as well. Put in everyday English you can say it means to want.

That would be my choice, to desire, is to want. So please allow me to go with want and desire interchangeably. When wanting or desire, if you will, is coupled with belief, a very powerful combination of elements is created but communication with the subconscious incomplete until you add the element of thought.

When these three powerful elements "Thought, Belief and Desire" are combined they create the most dynamic and magnificent, extraordinary and powerful force in the universe.

The subconscious mind; (AKA in my book "THE FORCES OF YOUR MIND" collectively I have named the three as one "THE FORCE").

When you wish to accomplish a particular activity no matter what or how difficult it may seem, or how many hard-ships you may encounter along the way and no matter how long it may take, if you think and stay focused believe in it and want it with every fiber of your being, you will most certainly achieve success.

There are some people who go through life expecting nothing and accepting whatever comes along, they take whatever they are given as though there was nothing else. In their own small way these people are satisfied and to a large extent they may even be called successful, because that's their world and that is the way they choose to live it.

And then there are those people who are the unsuccessful complainers. These people make silent wishes to themselves. I wish I had a new car, or I wish I could afford this or that, they may say. They go to sleep at night dreaming of a better life and wake in the morning to the same old unfulfilled wishes and desires but they never do anything to ever change their mundane monotonous boring lifestyle.

I am not poking fun at anyone. The point is you and only you can change your life. Having the misfortune of living without fulfillment of your desires should be sufficient reason enough for wanting to change.

Understand that you are not cemented to your environment. I am merely saying if you are not satisfied with the way things are In your life you have the power to change it.

Stop wishing and dreaming and do something about it. It's up to you. It's your life and you are the only one who can change it.

Life on earth is very short term. You start to realize that more and more as you get older. Everyone should try to live their lives to the fullest. You can change the way things are in your life; you can be a success at anything you desire but remember no one is going to hand success to you; it does take effort on your part. You really must want it.

As I said no one is going to hand it to you. You must take charge of your life and believe in yourself and go for the brass ring. I say you can be a success in everything and anything you do.

But just what is success? Success can be measured many different ways. Most people measure success by financial wealth, they do, I don't. Here's why.

Lots of people are financially wealthy. Often however, the money they have is the result of the hard work by others before them and they are simply lucky enough to be the recipient of a large estate and reap the benefits of the hard work by others through inheritance.

I say they are not successful people; they are lucky people to be the recipient of a financial treasure earned by the hard work of others who have past on.

Don't you agree and sometimes wish you had a very rich relative who left you their fortune. That would be nice but it's unlikely to happen to most of us.

My friend, wealth is not a true measure by which we attain success. Wealth can be one of the rewards we get sometimes when we are successful but more often than not we are successful when we accomplish a particular event that has concluded in a favorable desired result without any financial gain. So you see success can also be measured by favorable and desired accomplishments. That makes sense doesn't it?

Here are a couple of examples; remembering that success can mean different things to different people.

Example: A mountain climber reaches the highest peak (he thought himself or herself successful) because he or she continually thought about it and wanted to do it and believed that he or she could climb that mountain. It was quite an accomplishment, he or she was successful.

Example: A deep sea diver braves the depths of an ocean to bring up some ancient artifact and knows well in advance the artifact will be kept in a museum for others to see. His only compensation is the successful retrieval of the priceless article but is completely satisfied knowing that others will also enjoy viewing it.

Of course the examples above are individual ones, but often time's whole groups of people can be successful. A group of people help rebuild a neighbor's house that was lost in a storm. They succeeded to rebuild the house in record time without any monetary compensation, etc.

You can measure your own success, do it without the need of always thinking about cashing in.

Alright that's enough lessons on the English language of which few of us are expert. I am sure you fully understand by now how we measure success.

This book is about you and how you can lose weight through positive thinking so let's get back to talking about your success.

What is it you want out of your life? Do you believe whatever it is can be yours? Well, it can be yours if you want it bad enough.

Think it. Want it. Believe it. Whatever you choose if it is reasonable it can be yours. It's the law of the subconscious forces of the mind. The subconscious forces of your mind must and will satisfy every reasonable demand placed upon it by you. I have used a key word twice in the last two sentences, the key word of course is reasonable. Many of us wish for things to happen that are not reasonable and are unrealistic. An example of unreasonable and unrealistic wishful thinking would be perhaps, to wish your boss go to some very hot place when refusing to give you a raise in salary or time off for your birthday.

If it is reasonable and if you constantly think about it and really want it and believe in yourself, you will achieve whatever it is you desire.

Don't be fooled by the negativity of others who often make off hand or sly remarks that may let you feel you are wasting your time in your endeavor. In reality they don't want you to succeed. They want you to remain on their level. Misery loves company.

Remember they are the non-achievers, they wish and they dream about so many things they would like to have, yet they do little else to improve themselves. Stay clear of this group of negative thinkers if you can. Be your own person and never ever say you can't.

"Believe You Can And You Will"

Chapter 6: The Power Statement

An affirmation is a statement (and to use a few synonyms can also be confirmation, assertion, pronouncement, declaration, announcement, verification) of Truth consciously used so as to become the directing power of Life's expression."

To thoroughly understand the concept of the subconscious and the forces of your mind you must first believe, accept and understand that there are two distinct entities that are part of and live in the mind of every human being.

The names most given to these parts are the conscious mind and the subconscious mind. I described the important function of each of these entities at the beginning of this book. We talked about the important functions each of these entities play in our lives.

I briefly described the method by which the subconscious mind learns and ultimately uses to bring about a conscious desired result. In this chapter we will explore deeper into the needs of the subconscious mind, that it may hasten to bring about the reality of commands thrust upon it by the conscious mind.

It is human nature that we learn to do most everything by our senses, tasting, seeing, touching, smelling, hearing, and I'll add one more and that is by doing. Doing of course is not regarded as a natural sense. It may be considered and regarded as function of a person performing a specific task or deed. However, call it what you may, I believe doing, is as important as all of the other five senses. Doing combines a few of our natural senses in one.

The reason I make this conclusion is simple enough. The more often you do something, or anything, the easier it becomes. Haven't you found that to be true? Remember, practice makes perfect.

Of course doing it is not a natural human sense because it is not automatic and so we must make an effort to do whatever it is we are doing. But who can argue that the process of doing something repeatedly is not a powerful learning process.

We learn many things automatically through our natural human senses. We learn to recognize hundreds of different sounds and know what they are without actually seeing them. We see things and know what they are without touching them. We know what things should smell like without tasting. We know how things should taste without eating them. We know what things should feel like without touching them.

83

Our conscious mind accepts without question almost everything our senses provide to us as being true. If the use of any of our senses is used over and over in an action we soon believe the action to always be true even if it were not. Sometimes things are not what we think they should be.

I have experienced an example of this phenomenon from my training in the armed forces. For example the sweet smell of new mown grass; in World Wars One and Two and probably others, mustard gas was deliberately disguised to smell just like freshly cut grass. The senses could not detect the hidden danger and would treat this action as being truly the aroma of new mown grass.

However, the subconscious mind, being the master of all does not readily accept everything as being true as quickly as does the conscious mind. The subconscious mind requires more information before it becomes convinced the demands sent to it by the conscious mind are true.

However, the subconscious mind responds in kind only when it is convinced the conscious mind is not merely making another common frivolous wish. Remember, merely wishing for this or that doesn't work. If it did we would all be millionaires.

The subconscious mind responds to the repeated demands of the conscious mind. If more than one sense can be facilitated to expedite a particular result from the subconscious mind then by all means we should use as many of our senses that is practical.

If you're not quite sure of what I tried to convey in that last paragraph an example might help. Let's say for instance you want to lose weight, that's great; you purchased this book for that very reason and learned there is a verbal mantra in the last chapter that you can use to help you accomplish that worthy goal. You know you must repeat the verbal mantra a number of times for it to be absorbed by the subconscious mind.

We learned the subconscious mind will respond to the verbal commands of the conscious mind when it's convinced the conscious mind is not merely wishing.

If you were to use just my verbal mantra as written, the subconscious mind would eventually believe the demands being given to it and it would bring about your desired result. But this process of course does take time and seldom or rarely does the result you want happen overnight. There are some reports when desired results have been acquired miraculously over night but this is rare and should not be expected.

It is human nature to be impatient and most would give up trying to convince the subconscious mind to bring about their desired result because their desired results do not come fast enough. Giving up would be a terrible mistake, remember it probably took years to form and create the problem you have, trying to rid yourself of it overnight isn't fair to expect.

Depending upon the individual the time it takes to convince the subconscious mind to respond does of course vary. There is a way however to speed up the process and convince the subconscious mind to hasten a desired result. I call this process, the process of affirmation.

Affirmation simply means to declare a truth. I believe the practice of affirmations plays a very important part of positive thinking. Affirmations inform the subconscious mind that you are indeed very serious about your repeated demands and request desired results to come about as quickly as possible.

When more than one of our natural senses are used, it shortens the time it takes for the subconscious mind to produce a desired result. One way to accomplish this is by using affirmations.

I have listed below some definitions of the meaning of affirmation to help you more fully understand the meaning and the important part it plays in positive thinking and how it may be used to bring about your expected desired result from demands you give to the subconscious mind.

Affirmation refers primarily to the practice of positive thinking and the belief that a positive mental attitude supported by affirmations will achieve success in anything.

More specifically an affirmation is a carefully formatted statement that should be repeated to one's self as often as practical in the morning upon arising, through the day, and in the evening before sleep.

For an affirmation to be effective, it should be said in voice, kept as short and specific as possible and repeated as often as practical.

Affirmations are repeated positive statements that acknowledge life, said aloud or silently.

Affirmations reinforce the power of positive thinking.

Affirmations are simple short, powerful statements. When you say them or think them or even hear them, they become the thoughts that create your own reality.

Affirmations make you consciously aware of your thoughts. When you start making conscious positive thoughts, you remove negative thoughts.

Affirmations make you conscious of your thoughts. To affirm means to say something positively.

Affirmation means to declare firmly and assert something to be true.

Affirmations are statements where you assert that what you want to be true is true.

Affirmations are statements when made can affect the outcome of your life.

Positive affirmations are words of encouragement.

Affirmations will not work for anyone if the statements are lies.

Affirmations will work for anyone if the statements are the truth.

When the subconscious mind believes, its awesome power creates the reality of the affirmation.

Think it, desire it, believe it.

When we can combine more than one of our senses to convince the subconscious mind to bring about a desired result, the combination of senses serves to fortify the demands we consciously are making. An example would be to make use of a powerful affirmation using as many of our senses as is practical.

When using the force mantra, say the words aloud or silently but use your voice in addition to just reading the words to yourself, then by doing so we would be using our sense of sight as well as the sense of hearing. Because we are speaking the words as well as seeing the words, do you see where I am going with this idea of using as many of our senses as we can?

In the example above we used two of our five senses to help speed up the time it takes to convince our subconscious mind that our repeated demand for a desired result is really what we want.

We now know how we used the sense of sight as well as the sense of hearing? What if we were to add another sense? Well if we did, that would certainly hasten the time for the subconscious mind to act. We could add the sense of touch.

We add the sense of touch by using an old method of keeping tract of the number of times something is said, using the mechanics of counting knots tied and formed on a string, or beads, whatever is used doesn't matter; the method is ancient but practical and efficient. When we use this mechanical means of counting we add the sense of touching and it strengthens and hastens our demands.

This method is used by monks and many other groups of practitioners to help facilitate the number of times their mantra is being said.

"Believe You Can And You Will"

Chapter 7: The Positive Thinkers

"Only they can, who think they can!"

Confidence is the father of achievement. It reinforces ability, doubles energy, buttresses mental faculties, and increases power.

Your thought will carry only the force of your conviction, the weight of your decision, and the power of your confidence. If these are weak, your thought will be weak and your work futile. Some people are incapable of strong, deep conviction; they are all surface, and liable to be changed by the opinions of everyone else.

If they resolve upon a certain course, their resolution is so superficial that the first obstacle they strike deflects them. They are always at the mercy of the opposition, or of people who do not agree with them. Such people are shifty and unreliable; they lack strength of decision, of resolution.

What is a man good for if he hasn't strength of resolution? If his convictions are on the surface, he stands for nothing; nobody has confidence in him. He may be a good man, personally, but he does not inspire confidence.

No one would think of calling upon him when anything of importance was at stake. Unless

91

conviction takes hold of one's very being; there will be very little achievement in life.

It is the man whose conviction is rooted deep and takes hold of his very life-blood, the man who is strong and persistent in his determination that can be depended upon. He is the man of influence, who carries weight; he is above the influence of any man who happens to have a different opinion.

No one ever accomplishes anything in this world until he affirms in one way or another that he can do what he undertakes.

It is almost impossible to keep a man back who has a firm faith in his mission, who believes that he can do the thing before him, that he is equal to the obstacles which confront him, that he is more than a match for his environment.

The constant affirmation of ability to succeed, and of our determination to do so, carries us past difficulties, defies obstacles, laughs at misfortunes, and strengthens the power to achieve. It reinforces and buttresses the natural faculties and powers, and holds them to their tasks.

Constant affirmation increases courage, and courage is the backbone of confidence. Furthermore, when a person gets in a tight place and says, "I must," "I can," " I am" he not only reinforces his courage and strengthens his confidence, but also weakens the opposite qualities. Whatever strengthens a positive will weaken the corresponding negative.

You can do a difficult thing only with a positive state of mind, never with a negative. Plus force, not minus, does things. The dominant qualities are all positive, assertive, aggressive, and they require a corresponding attitude of mind for their exercise and application.

A man who has not these dominant qualities can never be a leader or independent; he must be a trailer, an imitator, until he changes his thought from negative to positive, from doubtful to certain, from shrinking and retiring to asserting and advancing. It is the decisive, positive soul that wins.

If you wish to amount to anything in the world, never for one moment permit the idea to come into your mind that you are unlucky, that you are less fortunate than other human beings. Deny it with all the power you can muster. Discipline yourself never to acknowledge weakness or think of mental, physical, or moral defects.

Deny that you are a weakling, that you cannot do what others can do; that you are handicapped and must be satisfied to take an inferior position in the world.

Strangle every doubt as you would a viper threatening your life. Never talk, think, or write of your poverty or unfortunate condition. Cut out of your life all thought that limits, hampers, dwarfs, and darkens it. These are ghosts of fear; the Creator never made them or intended them to haunt and torment you. He made you for happiness, for joy, for conquest over your environment.

Persistently affirm that the Creator handicapped no one, that our limitations are all our own. Resolve that, come what may, you will be an optimist; that there shall be nothing pessimistic in you; believe in the final triumph of the right, the victory of all that is true and noble.

Affirm that you are one of the most fortunate beings.

Congratulate yourself that you were born just in the nick of time, and in just the right place; that there is a definite work for you to do that no one else can do; and that you are one of the most lucky persons in the world to have the opportunity, the health, the education, to do the things you are bound to accomplish.

If you are out of work and poor, just throw out of your mind every idea of penury and poverty. Hold the thought of plenty, of abundance, of all good, which the Creator has promised you.

Stoutly deny that you are poor, or miserable, or unlucky; claim that you are well, vigorous, and strong; that you must succeed, and you will succeed.

Always affirm that the Creator, who gave you the longing to be somebody and to do something in the world, has also given you the ability and the opportunity to realize the ambition.

When you set your mind toward achievement, let everything about you indicate success. Let your manner, your dress, your bearing, your conversation, and everything you do speak achievement and success. Carry always a success atmosphere with you.

You will find a wonderful advantage in starting out every morning with the mind set toward success and achievement by permeating it with thoughts of prosperity and harmony, whether by repetition of set mantras, as some advise, or not. It will then be so much the harder for discord to get into the day's work.

If you are inclined to doubt your ability to do any particular thing, school yourself to hold the self-trust thought firmly and persistently. It is the assumption of power, of self-trust, of confidence in yourself, in your integrity or wholeness, that cannot be shaken, that will enable you to become strong, and to do, with vigor and ease, the thing you undertake.

You will find that the perpetual holding of these ideals will change your whole outlook upon life. You will approach your problems from a new standpoint, and life will take on a fresh meaning.

This perpetual affirmation will put you in harmony with your surroundings; it will make you contented and happy; and it will be a powerful tonic for your health. It will help you to build up individuality and personal power. It will make your brain clearer, your thought more effective. Keeping the mental machinery clean makes for vigorous thinking, decisive action.

If you are deficient in any quality, you can strengthen it by constant affirmation. If you are a coward anywhere in your nature (and most people are), you can strengthen courage by constantly affirming that you are absolutely fearless, that you are courageous, and that nothing can harm you.

Reason that fear is simply the sense of danger, and when you have perfect confidence in the great Creator's purpose, when you trust it implicitly, there will be no cause for fear.

If you have convinced yourself that there is only one great cause, that the opposite must be a delusion, you will gradually lose the sense of fear and gain the courage you desire.

Every time you feel a sense of fear come over you say: "I am absolutely fearless; there is nothing to fear; fear is not a reality; it is not the truth of being. It is only the absence of courage, based upon ignorance of the great cause."

Emerson knew the virtue of this philosophy when he said: "Nerve us with incessant affirmation. Don't bark against the bad, but chant the beauties of the good."

Stoutly determine not to harbor anything in the mind, which you do not wish to become real in your life. Shun poisoned thoughts, ideas that depress and make you unhappy, as instinctively as you avoid physical danger of any kind.

Do not entertain a discordant or an unhappy thought, or a thought of weakness and misery, but replace all these with cheerful, hopeful, optimistic thoughts.

When you feel out of sorts, blue, discouraged, disheartened, if you form the habit of suggesting to yourself some agreeable or pleasant subject, to dwell upon or think about, or take up some word or idea which will suggest pleasure, happiness, and harmony, you will be surprised to see how quickly you can change the whole course of your thought, and when this is changed, the feeling will change also.

You will increase your courage and confidence, and this is half the battle. You will soon find that your environment will begin to change. Hope will brighten and you will have a healthier outlook upon life. Then thought, instead of depressing your mind, will be a perpetual tonic of encouragement, and light will soon break and drive out the darkness.

All that you dream of, all that you yearn for and long to be, will be within your reach if you have the power to affirm sufficiently strong, if you can focus your faculties with sufficient intentness on a single purpose. It is concentration upon the thing you wish that brings it to you, whether it is health, money, or position.

Constantly affirm that which you wish, hold it persistently in the thought, concentrate all the power of you mind upon it, and when the mind is sufficiently positive and creative the desired thing will come to you as certainly as a stone

98

will come to the earth, when left free in the air, through the attracting influence of gravitation. You make yourself a magnet to draw the condition you wish.

"Man becomes what he believes", Anton Chekhov.

"Believe that life is worth living, and your belief will help create that fact", William James.

"Our belief at the beginning of a doubtful undertaking is the one thing that ensures the successful outcome of our venture", William James.

"We are what we believe we are", Benjamin N. Cardozo.

"If you constantly think of illness, you eventually become ill; if you believe yourself to be beautiful, you become so", Shakti Gawain.

"You have to believe in happiness, or happiness never comes", Douglas Malloch.

"If you keep on saying things are going to be bad, you have a good chance of being a prophet", Isaac Bashevis Singer.

"What one believes to be true either is true or becomes true within limits to be found experientially and experimentally. These limits are beliefs to be transcended", John Lilly.

"The thing always happens that you really believe in; and the belief in a thing makes it happen", Frank Lloyd Wright.

"The name we give to something shapes our attitude toward it", Katherine Paterson.

"If you think you can, you can. And if you think you can't, you're right", Mary Kay Ash.

"Man's rise or fall, success or failure, happiness or unhappiness depends on his attitude ... a man's attitude will create the situation he imagines", James Lane Allen.

"The greatest discovery of my generation is that man can alter his life simply by altering his attitude of mind", William James.

"Life has, indeed, many ills, but the mind that views every object in its most cheering aspect, and every doubtful dispensation as replete with latent good, bears within itself a powerful and perpetual antidote", Lydia H. Sigourney.

"Immense power is acquired by assuring yourself in your secret reveries that you were born to control affairs", Andrew Carnegie.

"Man's real life is happy, chiefly because he is ever expecting that it soon will be so", Edgar Allan Poe.

"I am optimistic and confident in all that I do. I affirm only the best for others and myself. I am the creator of my life and my world. I meet daily challenges gracefully and with complete confidence. I fill my mind with positive, nurturing, and healing thoughts", Alice Potter.

"Every thought we think is creating our future". Louise L. Hay

"The words "I am ..." are potent words; be careful what you hitch them to". "The thing you're claiming has a way of reaching back and claiming you", A. L. Kitselman

"Self-image sets the boundaries of individual accomplishment", Maxwell Maltz.

"Nothing can stop the man with the right mental attitude from achieving his goal; nothing on earth can help the man with the wrong mental attitude", WW. Ziege.

"They can because they think they can", Virgil.

"Life is a mirror and will reflect back to the thinker what he thinks into it", Ernest Holmes.

"Our minds can shape the way a thing will be because we act according to our expectations", Federico Fellini.

"A man is literally what he thinks"; James Lane Allen.

"The happiness of your life depends upon the quality of your thoughts ... take care that you entertain no notions unsuitable to virtue and reasonable nature", Marcus Aurelius.

"You cannot escape the results of your thoughts.... Whatever your present environment may be, you will fall, remain or rise with your thoughts, your vision, and your ideal". "You will become as small as your controlling desire, as great as your dominant aspiration", James Lane Allen.

"The life each of us lives is the life within the limits of our own thinking. To have life more abundant, we must think in limitless terms of abundance", Thomas Dreier.

"A man's life is what his thoughts make it", Marcus Aurelius.

"You create yourself in the image you hold in your mind", Thomas Dreier.

"A man is what he thinks about all day long", Ralph Waldo Emerson.

"All that we are is the result of what we have thought". "The mind is everything. What we think, we become", Buddha.

"Think you can, think you can't; either way, you'll be right", Henry Ford.

"Our destiny changes with our thoughts; we shall become what we wish to become, do what we wish to do, when our habitual thoughts correspond with our desires", Orison Swett Marden.

"Our best friends and our worst enemies are our thoughts. A thought can do us more good than a doctor or a banker or a faithful friend. It can also do us more harm than a brick", Dr. Frank Crane.

"The way a man's mind runs is the way he is sure to go", Henry B. Wilson.

"The soul contains the event that shall befall it, for the event is only the actualization of its thoughts, and what we pray to ourselves for is always granted", Ralph Waldo Emerson.

"As you think, you travel, and as you love, you attract. You are today where your thoughts have brought you; you will be tomorrow where your thoughts take you", James Lane Allen.

"God will help you if you try, and you can if you think you can", Anna Delaney Peale.

"To expect defeat is nine-tenths of defeat itself", Francis Marion Crawford.

"The quality of our expectations determines the quality of our action", Andre Godin.

"What a man thinks of himself, that is what determines, or rather indicates his fate" Henry David Thoreau.

"Man, being made reasonable, and so a thinking creature, there is nothing more worthy of his being than the right direction and employment of his thoughts; since upon this depends both his usefulness to the public, and his own present and future benefit in all respects", William Penn.

"Great men are they who see that the spiritual is stronger than any material force, that thoughts rule the world", Ralph Waldo Emerson.

"Never think any oldish thoughts. Its oldish thoughts that make a person old", James A. Farley.

"As a man thinketh, so is he, as a man chooseth, so is he.

"Thoughts lead on to purposes; purposes go forth in action; actions form habits; habits decide character; and character fixes our destiny", Tyron Edwards.

"Keep your thoughts right, for as you think, so are you. Therefore, think only those things that will make the world better, and you unashamed", Henry H. Buckley.

"Every man is free to rise as far as he's able or willing, but the degree to which he thinks determines the degree to which he'll rise". Ayn Rand.

"What you think means more than anything else in your life", George Matthew Adams.

"Change your thoughts and you change your world", Norman Vincent Peale.

"The way in which we think of ourselves has everything to do with how our world sees us", Arlene Raven.

"Be careful of your thoughts; they may become words at any moment", Ira Gassen.

"The wisdom of all ages and cultures emphasizes the tremendous power our thoughts have over our character and circumstances", Liane Cordes.

"We are never so happy or as unhappy as we think", Francois de La Rochefoucauld.

"Man is only miserable so far as he thinks himself so", Jacopo Sannazaro.

"A man's as miserable as he thinks he is", Marcus Annaeus Seneca.

"The most unhappy of all men is he who believes himself to be so", David Hume.

"The mind is its own place, and in itself can make a heaven of hell, a hell of heaven", John Milton.

"All happiness is in the mind" .

"Happiness is not a matter of events, it depends upon the tides of the mind", Alice Meynell.

"I am happy and content because I think I am", Alain-Rene Lesage.

"A happy life consists in tranquility of mind", Cicero.

"The happiest person is the person who thinks the most interesting thoughts", William Lyon Phelps.

"Unhappiness indicates wrong thinking, just as ill health indicates a bad regimen", Paul Bourget.

"Happiness does not depend on outward things, but on the way we see them", Leo Tolstoy.

"Happiness will never be any greater than the idea we have of it", Maurice Maeterlinck.

"Misery is almost always the result of thinking", Joseph Joubert.

"Some patients I see are actually draining into their bodies the diseased thoughts of their minds", Zachary T. Bercovitz.

"The body manifests what the mind harbors", Jerry Augustine.

"Since the human body tends to move in the direction of its expectations-plus or minus-it is important to know that attitudes of confidence and determination are no less a part of the treatment program than medical science and technology", Norman Cousins.

"You can promote your healing by your thinking", James E. Sweeney.

"Most of the time we think we're sick it's all in the mind", Thomas Wolfe.

"The pessimist is half-licked before he starts", Thomas A. Buckner.

"No one can defeat us unless we first defeat ourselves", Dwight D. Eisenhower.

"You live with your thoughts-so be careful what they are", Eva Arrington.

"We must dare to think unthinkable thoughts", James W. Fulbright.

"Thoughts have power; thoughts are energy". "And you can make your world or break it by your own thinking", Susan Taylor.

"Your imagination has much to do with your life. It is for you to decide how you want your imagination to serve you", Philip Conley.

"I cannot discover that anyone knows enough to say definitely what is and what is not possible", Henry Ford.

"A human being fashions his consequences as surely as he fashions his goods or his dwelling. Nothing that he says, thinks or does is without consequences", Norman Cousins.

"We create our fate every day; most of the ills we suffer from are directly traceable to our own behavior", Henry Miller.

"We choose our joys and sorrows long before we experience them", Kahlil Gibran.

"Man does not simply exist, but always decides what his existence will be, what he will become in the next moment", Viktor Frankl.

"The principle of life is that life responds by corresponding; your life becomes the thing you have decided it shall be", Raymond Charles Barker.

"We are accountable only to ourselves for what happens to us in our lives", Mildred Newman.

"If you keep saying things are going to be bad, you have a good chance of being a prophet", Isaac Bashevis Singer.

"Whatsoever a man soweth, that shall he also reap", Bible.

"If a man plants melons he will reap melons; if he sows beans, he will reap beans", Chinese proverb.

"A person who doubts himself is like a man who would enlist in the ranks of his enemies and bear arms against himself". "He makes his failure certain by himself being the first person to be convinced of it", Alexandre Dumas.

109

"To be ambitious for wealth, and yet always expecting to be poor; to be always doubting your ability to get what you long for, is like trying to reach east by traveling west".

"There is no philosophy that will help a man to succeed when he is always doubting his ability to do so, and thus attracting failure".

"No matter how hard you work for success, if your thought is saturated with the fear of failure, it will kill your efforts, neutralize your endeavors and make success impossible", Charles Baudouin.

"He who fears being conquered is sure of defeat", Napoleon Bonaparte.

"Treat people as if they were what they should be, and you help them become what they are capable of becoming", Johann von Goethe.

"People have a way of becoming what you encourage them to be-not what you nag them to be", S. N. Parker.

"Our self-image, strongly held, essentially determines what we become", Maxwell Maltz

"Act as if it were impossible to fail", Dorothea Brande.

"If you want a quality, act as if you already had it". William James

"If you would be powerful, pretend to be powerful", Home Tooke.

"If one advances confidently in the direction of his dreams, and endeavors to live the life, which he has imagined, he will meet with a success unexpected in common hours", Henry David Thoreau.

"We are what we pretend to be, so we must be careful about what we pretend to be", Kurt Vonnegut.

"Act as if you were already happy, and that will tend to make you happy", Dale Carnegie.

"We become just by performing just actions, temperate by performing temperate actions, brave by performing brave actions", Aristotle.

"If you act like you're rich, you'll get rich", Adnan Koashoggi.

"It is never too late to be what you might have been", George Eliot.

"The only prison we need to escape from is the prison of our own minds".

"He was a "how" thinker, not an "if" thinker".

"This I conceive to be the chemical function of humor: to change the character of our thought", Lin Yutang.

"The young do not know enough to be prudent, and therefore they attempt the impossible-and achieve it, generation after generation", Pearl S. Buck.

"Believe You Can And You Will"

Notes: